Vision of the Miracle

By

Carolyn C Marks

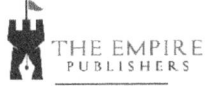

12808 West Airport Blvd Suite 270M Sugar Land, TX 77478, Unites States

https://www.theempirepublishers.com/

Our books may be purchased in bulk for promotional, educational, or business use.

Please contact The Empire Publishers at +1 844 636-4579, or by email at support@theempirepublishers.com

First Edition December 2025

About the Author

"Vision of The Miracle" was written with one purpose in mind: to glorify God. While I can't share everything, I will do my best to offer a glimpse of the journey. Sister Carolyn Marks, a woman of unwavering faith, was born on a farm in Caroline County and raised in the small town of Ashland, Virginia. This memoir had to be written because my testimony is too powerful to keep to myself. It is vital to share our stories to inspire others, to offer hope, healing, and to be living witnesses of God's grace. I firmly believe that God allows certain trials to test our character and strengthen our faith. As a mother, grandmother, daughter, retired banker, retired school teacher, and now, a writer, my devotion to faith and family shines brightly. Each chapter of my life has been shaped by God's hand, and I am excited to invite you to join me on this faith-filled journey. Come, walk with me in faith.

Dedication

To God be the glory for the great things He has done! His grace and love have been my guiding light throughout this journey. Indeed, He has done marvelous things!

A unique and heartfelt "Thank You" to my late, beloved father. His wisdom and unwavering faith shaped the person I am today. I will never forget his words: "Sugar, you must be born again," as he gently encouraged me to give my life to Christ. He lived the truth before us all, and his example remains a cornerstone of my faith.

To my dearly beloved mother, thank you for your love, support, and guidance throughout this memoir. Your strength, wisdom, and tireless work ethic have inspired me in more ways than I can express. You managed eight of us— four boys and four girls—with grace, patience, and a heart full of love. Ninety-three years later, you still smile, making it all look easy. I am truly blessed to be your child.

I am deeply grateful to my family for their unwavering support. My daughter stood by my side throughout this journey, and my son and their father were also there for me. Your love and encouragement have meant the world to me.

To my Beloved Pastor and his wife, your spiritual guidance and prayers have been invaluable. Thank you for your love. Thank you for walking with me in faith and for your constant support. A special thanks to Minister Burnett, whose help in choosing a title was greatly appreciated.

This book is a reflection of the love, faith, and guidance I have received from all of you. I am forever grateful.

Table of Contents

The Beginning of My Journey

I wasn't born with a silver spoon in my mouth and my upbringing was anything but glamorous. I grew up in the small town of Ashland, VA., where life was simple but never easy. My parents were hard-working people. They had to be, with eight children—four girls and four boys—to care for. We didn't have much, but we had enough. Their work ethic and love for their family built a foundation that carried us through even tough times.

My father was a profoundly religious man, a Jehovah's Witness who served as an Elder in the congregation. As a child, I witnessed his devotion. His faith wasn't just something he practiced; it was his way of life. He poured himself into his role in the Kingdom Hall, guiding others and raising us in a strict yet loving spiritual environment. My siblings and I grew up surrounded by faith, attending meetings regularly and following the teachings he held dear. At that time, I believed nothing could shake my father's faith. He was so committed, so sure.

But as life often teaches us, even the strongest can falter. He discovered that, like all people, the Jehovah Witnesses were flawed. Their shortcomings began weighing on him, leading to a profound disillusionment. It wasn't long before he started questioning everything he had been so dedicated to. The realization that Jehovah's Witnesses were not perfect people hit him hard, and he struggled to reconcile his faith with this newfound understanding.

My father, the man I had always known to be unwavering in his beliefs, began to drift away from God. It was as if the disillusionment had unmoored him, setting him in doubt. Eventually, he left the Kingdom Hall altogether. The man who had once been an Elder, guiding others, found himself wandering. He turned to the streets, seeking solace in things he never would have. He began drinking, womanizing, and engaging in behaviors entirely out of character for him. It was painful to watch his decline, to see the man we had looked up to for so long lose his way.

During that difficult time, I often wondered if we would ever get the man we knew back. But God has a way of stepping in when all seems lost. My father's redemption came from an unexpected source—his sister, my aunt. She was a member of Refuge Church of Our Lord Jesus Christ, a Holiness church, in Sandston Va..She e never gave up on him. She witnessed to him tirelessly, sharing her faith and reminding him that God's love and grace were still there for him. Little by little, her words began to penetrate his heart.

One day, something in my father shifted. He realized that God was still reaching out to him no matter how far he had fallen. He repented his sins and made the life-changing decision to return to God. He was drawn to Refuge, where my aunt attended. He was baptized in the name of the Lord Jesus Christ and received the Holy Ghost, speaking in tongues as the Spirit gave him utterance. The transformation was nothing short of a miracle.

My father became a completely different man—he was born again. The things he had once done, the streets he had turned to, all faded away. He stopped drinking, stopped living the way he had when he'd drifted from God, and became a living testimony to the power of faith and redemption. His dedication to his new faith was inspiring, and soon, his enthusiasm spilled over into our family. He couldn't stop witnessing to us, sharing his story, and urging us to experience the same grace that had changed his life.

At that time, my family and I were fellowshipping at a local Baptist church. As my father's faith grew, he invited us. He wanted us to come with him to Refuge to see the transformation in his life. First, my mother visited. She was moved by what she saw, and before long, she was baptized and saved. My sister followed soon after, finding her own spiritual home in Refuge.

My father didn't stop there—he continued to invite me. I had seen his changes, and while I was curious, I wasn't quite ready to take that step. But one Sunday, everything changed. I had planned to attend Union Baptist Church as usual. I was driving the familiar route when I approached a fork in the road. If I veered right, I would go to Ashland and my Baptist church, as I always did. But as my hand began to turn the wheel, something extraordinary happened.

A quickening came into my right arm, almost like a gentle force nudging me in a different direction. Instead of turning toward Ashland, my hand straightened out, and I continued driving straight ahead. That road led to 295S and eventually to Refuge Church in Sandston. At that moment, I knew the Lord was leading me somewhere new. It was clear that this wasn't just a coincidence; this was divine guidance, a call to see what was happening at Refuge.

When I walked into Refuge Church for the first time, the atmosphere was unlike anything I had ever experienced. It was my first time in a Holiness church, and the energy in the room was electric. The level of praise was unlike anything I had known. At my Baptist church, worship was quiet and reserved. Even the children were caught up in the Spirit, shouting "Hallelujah" repeatedly in loud, joyful voices. The contrast was striking, and I could feel God's presence in an almost tangible way.

I immediately felt the pull to be baptized, but on that day, there wasn't any water in the pool. I left, but the desire didn't fade. I returned soon after, determined to be baptized, and I was. On 23 June 1989, I received the Holy Ghost, as written in Acts 2:38-41. It was a moment that forever changed the course of my life. I had been touched by the same grace that had transformed my father, and there was no turning back.

From that day on, I became a member of Refuge, with the late Bishop Algenor Johnson as my pastor. Looking back now, I can see how God's hand guided me, just as it had guided my father. God was always leading us home through his fall and redemption through my moments of doubt and divine intervention.

My father's story and my own are reminders that no matter how far we wander, God is always waiting to welcome us back. He works in ways we don't always understand, but his love and grace are constant. And sometimes, all it takes is a quickening in the arm, a nudge in the right direction, to find ourselves on the path we were always meant to walk.

A Faith Walk

Hebrew 11:1 KJV Now faith is the substance of things hoped for, the evidence of things not seen.

In the transformative year of Y2K, God called me out of Refuge Sandston, leading me to cross paths with a Apostle from an Evangelistic Ministry. This wasn't your typical church fellowship—his ministry took place within the humble walls of his home, where faith was deep, and the Word of God was shared with profound precision.

Gone were the days of simply leaving your bible on the church pew after service. This ministry reshaped our relationship with scripture. *We learned what it meant to "study to show ourselves approved" (2 Tim 2:15),* to dive deeply, dissect, and understand God's Word in ways we had never understood. Hours would pass, yet the time felt sacred as we delved into scripture, prayer, and worship.

It was here that we embraced the whole Communion of believers. In each gathering, we prayed fervently, took Communion, washed one another's feet in acts of humility, and broke bread—living out the gospel in both word and deed. Every moment in those fellowships was a journey, binding us closer to God and one another in ways that still shape my faith today.

Let me take you back to August 2002—a day that began like any other but would change my life forever. It was a worship service, filled with the familiar rhythm of praise and prayer, yet something was indescribable in the air that day. As I joined in, surrounded by the warmth of my community, I felt a sense of anticipation, as if the very atmosphere was charged with a divine presence.

As the service progressed, I closed my eyes, surrendering wholly, and that's when something extraordinary happened. It started as a gentle tingling around me, an almost tangible energy that grew stronger, wrapping around me like a warm embrace. And then I was slain in the spirit. As clearly as if someone was lying beside me, I heard a voice. It wasn't the voice of the Apostle or someone nearby; the voice was a voice that echoed deep within my spirit—a voice unlike any I had ever heard before. It was small, quiet, firm, comforting, and filled with authority and love.

"I am the Lord that healeth thee," the voice declared, resonating in every fiber of my being. "I have healed your body. When you go home, throw your medicine away. Even if you have the signs or symptoms, you are healed." Exodus 15:26.

I lay there, stunned, as the words sank in. I had been battling a thyroid condition for some time, and my medication was part of my daily routine. I had grown accustomed to the pills and the regular doctor visits that kept my condition in check. But here I was, hearing something so powerful, so absolute, that I knew it was not an ordinary moment. This was God Himself, speaking directly to me. I felt peace and clarity like nothing I'd ever experienced.

The Apostle, standing nearby, seemed to sense what had just happened. His gaze met mine, filled with a deep understanding that only comes from years of spiritual wisdom. "You heard from God, didn't you?" he asked and his eyes reflecting a kindness and knowledge that mirrored my own.

I nodded, my heart pounding with awe yet feeling an inexplicable peace. The Apostle offered a gentle smile and gave me his blessing and words of encouragement that strengthened my resolve. As I left the sanctuary, a sense of purpose filled me, a certainty that I had received a divine promise of healing.

When I arrived home, I saw my medication on the kitchen counter—a familiar part of my daily routine. But today was different. I looked at those bottles, symbols of my reliance on earthly remedies, and knew I had a choice. I took a deep breath, gathered up the pills, and discarded them, feeling a mix of exhilaration and trepidation. I was stepping out in faith, trusting fully in the words I had heard, placing my health and my future in God's hands.

The days that followed were filled with both peace and challenge. My symptoms didn't immediately vanish, and at times, the temptation to go back to my medication was almost overwhelming. Doubts crept in, whispering questions that tested the strength of my conviction. But each time those doubts arose, I returned to that moment in the service, remembering the words spoken over me. In my quiet moments of prayer, I felt His presence, a steady reassurance that I was not alone. Each time I considered reaching for a remedy, I chose to wait on the Lord instead, leaning on the promise I had received.

In those days, my relationship with God deepened profoundly. I spent hours in prayer, meditating on His promises, and reading Scriptures that spoke of His healing power and steadfast love. I found myself drawn to passages describing His faithfulness, care for each of us, and boundless grace. Each verse was like a balm, a reminder that my healing journey was not just physical but spiritual. I began to see this experience as an invitation to draw closer to God and to trust Him completely.

Weeks turned into months, and my resolve was tested many times. Some days were easier than others, but through it all, I held firmly to the belief that healing was happening, even if I couldn't see it with my own eyes. Each lingering symptom became less a source of fear and more a symbol of my commitment to walk by faith. It was a journey of learning to trust, letting go of my need for immediate proof, and embracing the unseen work of the Great Physician.

During this journey, I understood that faith isn't always about seeing immediate results. Sometimes, it's about holding on to a promise, even when circumstances suggest otherwise. It's about believing in the One greater than our doubts and fears. My days were filled with conversations with God, moments where I would share my worries and listen for His gentle reassurance. I discovered that healing often goes beyond the physical; it's about aligning our hearts and minds with His love and purpose.

As time passed, I began to notice subtle changes. My symptoms grew less pronounced, and I felt a newfound energy and peace. It was as though God was slowly restoring me from the inside out, healing my body and spirit. Through every challenge, I found a growing confidence in His plan and a sense of calm that carried me through the most challenging days. And each day, I was reminded that faith is not a one-time decision but a continuous journey, a daily choice to trust.

This journey brought me into a deeper relationship with God than I had ever known before. I learned to rely on His strength, to find solace in His promises, and to trust in

His timing. I came to see that His ways are higher than ours and that sometimes He calls us to walk paths that challenge us so we can experience His love and grace in ways we never could otherwise.

As I look back on that day in August, I realize that it was the beginning of a new chapter in my life—a chapter defined by faith, healing, and a deeper understanding of God's unfailing love. This experience forever changed me; my faith strengthened, and my spirit renewed. And so, as I share this story, I hope it encourages those facing their own struggles. Know that there is a God who hears, who heals, and who walks with us through every trial.

It is just the beginning of my testimony—a testament to God's faithfulness and the transformative power of His love. For anyone reading this, may my journey be a reminder that in the arms of the Almighty Father, there is healing, restoration, and peace.

I Have a Testimony

Before I took my first breath, my soul had walked this earth, embraced by friendships, laughter, and life's flavors. Yet, none of it brought true fulfillment until the day I answered the call to faith—a call that gave me new life. Before that moment, I lived in an illusion of perfection, feeling nothing could add to my happiness. But deep down, this life was emptying me, pulling me away from what mattered most, leaving me a person who doubted, who had forgotten what faith felt like.

Then, God extended His hand in a moment that was as ordinary as life-changing. It was an invitation, a pathway to peace and purpose, and I accepted it with relief and joy. I sensed this was the turning point I'd needed, the one that would guide me out of worry and into a place of enduring comfort. Yet, let me tell you—this path of faith is not an easy road. It challenges, it demands, and it reveals. Faith, after all, is a journey that tests us, showing whether our beliefs stand firm or waver in the face of life's storms. The world tempts us, pulling us toward things that only offer temporary satisfaction. But for believers, the challenge is to hold steady, to stay unbroken on the path that leads to truth.

Faith is believing without seeing and trusting without knowing the outcome. It requires the strength to persist, even when others doubt. The journey of faith means defying the world's expectations and walking forward even when every voice tells you to turn back. Those who stay close to God in these times are the ones who understand that beyond the trials, there lies peace. **As God reminds us, "Come out from among them and be separate... touch no unclean thing, and I will receive you." (2 Corinthians 6:17)**

True righteousness demands we leave behind the world's empty promises and turn away from worshipping lesser things. Only by emptying ourselves of these distractions can we fully open our hearts to God. He, who created us, knows the weight of the world's lures and whispers. And He knows that not everyone will answer the call of faith—it requires dedication and a heart that seeks truth.

I once wandered, lost in my disbelief, but once I understood that my life was incomplete without God, everything changed. My days became filled with prayer, fasting, and the light of His wisdom. Those sleepless nights of worry were replaced by calm, by a peace that only faith could bring. I learned that God rewards those who hold steady and abandon worldly pursuits to pleasing the Creator. The road ahead often seemed daunting, but with each challenge, I trusted that if God led me to it, He would lead me through it. This mindset allowed me to scale mountains I once thought insurmountable.

God has the power to move mountains with a single word. Every grain of sand, every star obeys His will. He could wipe everything away in an instant, but He sustains the world with care, giving us chance after chance to find our way back to Him. No matter how often we stray or ignore His presence, He waits patiently, giving us endless opportunities to turn back and see the truth. When we finally look beyond ourselves, we see that the darkness surrounding us is often of our own making, a consequence of choices that lead us away from Him. But even then, God doesn't abandon us. He offers us a path to healing and a chance to rediscover the purpose that lights our souls.

The walk of faith saved me from the darkness that had surrounded me for so long. I tried countless times to break free from the things that weighed on my heart, but every attempt seemed to fall short. Only when I surrendered fully, asking God for strength and guidance, did I feel the grip of negativity loosen. In prayer, day and night, I found solace. I found God's hand and promised myself I would never again doubt Him. He is the one who truly knows me, has seen every struggle, and has loved me through it all. And with that love, I have found a life that was always meant to be—filled with purpose, faith, and the unwavering peace of walking by His side.

Jehovah Rapha Is My Doctor

There are countless paths we can walk in life. Differences are accepted and celebrated in a world that celebrates free will, self-expression, and the right to choose any direction. However, as inspiring as this freedom is, it sometimes pulls us away from our true purpose, leading us astray from the life God intended for us. He created us as imperfect beings, yet with purpose, and blessed us with the Holy Bible—a guide to living fully, honestly, and meaningfully. Its wisdom isn't apparent to everyone, but it opens doors to understanding, fulfillment, and peace to those who seek it sincerely.

We are all unique, carrying our beliefs and views. Embracing each other's differences brings harmony, but life without direction can lead to confusion, emptiness, and sometimes pain. The world offers countless alluring choices, yet when these paths stray from God, they often leave us feeling lost. I've encountered many lives, each with its ways and perspectives. Yet, each encounter taught me something: true peace lies not in the world's promises but in God's embrace. When I finally surrendered to His guidance, my worries melted away. I found a new strength, a sense of security, knowing the One who knows all was guiding me.

With time, I focused less on worldly distractions and more on God's voice. My days became dedicated to prayer, reflection, and aligning my heart with His Word. The more I surrendered, the clearer my purpose became—to share His message of hope and redemption. I joined an Evangelist Ministry, and on weekends, we stood on street corners in Washington, D.C., led by the spirit, reaching out to souls in need of light. The preachers would speak, and we, the sisters, would share our testimonies with those who'd listen. We visited churches, sharing the greatness of God, each story a reflection of His endless love and mercy.

I wanted to become a living example of Christ's love, to show others the peace and joy that faith brings. To guide others to the truth, you must embody it yourself. Through my actions and the calm faith placed upon my face, I hoped to reflect God's love, convincing people to embrace a life of purpose, joy, and truth rather than one of fleeting pleasures and hidden pain.

My heart aches when I see people weighed down by the world, their tired eyes, and weary souls searching for an escape. I know firsthand how the glittering promises of the world tempt us, only to leave us emptier than before. The Lord warned us of these deceptions, of the misery they bring. Yet, we often remain blind, grasping at false promises.

It can be terrifying to abandon the world's way and live by God's truth. We fear losing friends, family, and acceptance. But obeying the One who created it all won't lead to loss—it leads to a genuine connection with people who will stand by us on our faith journey. Faith in God provides the comfort that He never will, no matter who may leave. His guidance and His presence remain through every trial.

The secret to unlocking true power and peace in our lives is surrendering entirely to God. When we do, we experience the power of His Word, the cleansing of His Blood, the strength of the Holy Spirit, and the assurance of prayer. I have traveled to churches, sharing my testimony and proclaiming what God has done for me. I am overwhelmed by His mercy, which has transformed my life in ways words cannot fully capture. He saw my hidden pain, healed the wounds I could not heal, and removed every source of darkness.

I found freedom from the burdens I had carried for so long with God. His light replaced my struggles, His wisdom replaced my doubts, and His love replaced my fears. He gave me answers I didn't even know I was seeking, lifting me out of confusion and clarity. When I surrendered to Him, He gave me not just life but a life with purpose, joy, and an unbreakable faith.

The Joy of My Salvation

"For I will restore health unto thee, and I will heal thee of thy wounds, saith the Lord." — Jeremiah 30:17

We are not crafted as flawless beings; each day offers a new opportunity to grow, strengthen our faith, and align more closely with our Creator's plan. But we can't do it alone. God's wisdom and power sustain our lives—He alone knows what we truly need and delivers blessings beyond our understanding in His time.

Sometimes, faith can move mountains. When we think nothing will change, God opens new doors. But while we often hurry to find quick fixes, God sees the bigger picture and knows when the time is right. He is attuned to our every thought and feeling, knowing our desires and the struggles that burden us.

There was a time when I, like many others, was caught in the shadows of illness. It wasn't just physical but affected my spirit, outlook, and energy. Simple tasks felt like mountains, and days blurred from morning to night as I lay in bed, unable to move forward. Well-meaning people offered solutions—doctors, treatments, advice—but each time I considered them, something inside held me back. I felt a heaviness, an unexplainable pull to turn inward rather than out. I realized the answer was a deeper surrender to God, not human remedies.

My illness was quiet and often invisible to others, yet it changed everything. Life lost its shine, and each day felt like a shadow of what had been. As weeks turned to months, I felt no relief. Then, one day, my heart whispered what I had ignored: lay it all before God. I surrendered my pain, pouring out my struggles, worries, and every ache in prayer. The peace that followed was indescribable.

"Many are the afflictions of the righteous, but the LORD will deliver him out of them all." — Psalm 34:19

Whenever I felt afflicted, I turned to God with unwavering faith. In times of fever, I anointed myself, prayed with conviction, and watched as God restored me. My God can do anything, and this journey has taught me the unshakable power of faith. Whether it was high blood pressure or a simple cold, I asked Him to take it from me so I could continue sharing His light with others. Each time, He answered. No matter the time or place, God answered without hesitation, giving me strength when no one else could.

Unlike human relationships, where we sometimes fear judgment or rejection, God's mercy is infinite. People can judge quickly, often harshly, and indifferent to our struggles. But God listens. He is the ever-present comforter, open to our cries and quick to send peace. When we come to

Him with true faith and pure intentions, His healing touch is unmatched by any earthly cure.

God has assured us of His power to heal and restore, but we must approach Him with genuine, unwavering belief. When we pray with conviction, believing in His ability to solve even the most complex problems, we open the door to miracles. He waits patiently for us to seek His guidance and realize that only His path leads to true peace.

No doctor, no cure is more powerful than God's mercy. If we find ourselves in difficulty, it's a moment for growth, strengthening our faith, and turning fully to Him. Every trial is under His control, and the cure is as close as our prayers. God's love surpasses human love; He knows us better than we know ourselves.

When we finally lay our burdens at His feet, trusting in His divine care, we find the strength to rise. God's love is limitless, His mercy boundless, and with Him, there is always healing, always hope. In surrendering to Him, we unlock the peace, strength, and purpose that only He can provide.

Exceptional Job

There's a captivating allure to the world's promises, a glimmer of satisfaction that draws us in, no matter how hard we resist. But when these desires take over, overshadowing what truly matters, they often lead us further from our real purpose. It's easy to lose sight of the eternal joy God intended, exchanging lasting peace for the fleeting spark of worldly allure.

In June of 1989, God pulled me from my self-destruction. He reached into my life, full of mistakes and turmoil, and saved me with a love that went beyond my sins. Through His mercy, I received the precious gift of the Holy Ghost. It transformed me, igniting a drive to live for Christ—a life of light, love, and purpose. In August of 2002, I heard God's call again, anchoring me deeper in faith. Since then, I have run this race with Him, striving to be a beacon of hope, a reminder to others of the peace God brings.

I knew then that my purpose was to serve, to be a vessel for those seeking a way out of darkness. And God, in His grace, led me to live this purpose in ways I could never have planned. I took on various roles, one of the most cherished being a teaching assistant at Byrd Middle School. Despite my son's initial hesitation about the school, God had other plans. I was offered a position in the Exceptional Education Department, working one-on-one with a student with a disability (autism). It was an opportunity I embraced wholeheartedly, knowing that this was where God needed me to be.

For two beautiful years, I walked the halls of Byrd Middle School, sharing space with my children and guiding young minds. I had my little classroom, a reading room, where I connected with students profoundly. We learned, laughed, and grew together, and I saw God's creation in each child. Their purity, curiosity, and boundless spirit touched me deeply. Every morning, kids would wait at my door, sharing simple requests that reminded me of the power of small gestures. They relied on me, trusted me, and, in return, made me a better person.

But God's plan didn't end there. Encouraged by the school's principal, I pursued a teaching certification, earned a provisional license, and embarked on an unforgettable journey. In July 2006, I interviewed for a teaching position with Henrico County Public Schools. However, as a career switcher, I lacked traditional experience. But I knew how to pray, and so did those who supported me. On July 12, my prayers were answered—I was offered a teaching position at Highland Springs. Then, on September 5, 2006, I walked into my first official classroom, overwhelmed with gratitude.

Highland Springs was a Title One school, where most students were on free or reduced lunch. Though I lived on the other side of town, God placed me here, right where I was needed. As a teacher, I worked harder than ever, pouring my heart into my students. God blessed me with a room; the principal even supported a morning prayer group. Teachers gathered in unity, sharing strength through prayer. As I've learned, prayer changes things, and each day, I walk into my classroom, renewed by God's presence.

"Therefore, I tell you, whatever you ask in prayer, believe that you have received it, and it will be yours." — Mark 11:24

Teaching wasn't just a job—it was my mission field. It was just my students, God, and me within those four walls. We shared more than lessons; we shared life. We laughed, cried, and learned together, creating a bond built on trust and love. Many of my students just needed someone to care, to show them that they were seen, valued, and loved. I came to work every day ready to give one hundred and ten percent, knowing that even the smallest act of kindness could leave a lasting impact.

Through this journey, I became a different person—more compassionate, more resilient, and more grateful for the life God had given me. His love had lifted me from the depths and led me on a path I could never have imagined. Looking back, I see each step as a thread in the beautiful tapestry God has woven into my life. He taught me that true joy isn't found in the world's promises but His unending grace. God offers us abundant life through countless blessings, and those who are willing to open our hearts to His plan are the ones who truly live.

ReTired!

"Come to Me, All Who Labor and Are

Heavy Laden, and I Will Give You Rest."

Matthew 11:28

Embracing change is one of life's most complex challenges, especially when it means walking away from something you've poured your heart and soul into when your job becomes more than a paycheck and instead transforms into a calling, a mission, a reflection of your purpose, stepping away can feel like leaving behind a part of yourself. The routines, the triumphs, the challenges—all of it weaves into your identity. So, the void left behind can feel immeasurable.

Work often isn't just a job; it's a tapestry of meaning woven with purpose and passion. Letting go of that sense of meaning can be intimidating. The uncertainty of what lies ahead and the grief of leaving behind years of dedication can weigh heavily. But sometimes, when personal well-being is at stake, prioritizing yourself becomes an act of bravery.

June 2019 was a date etched in my mind. After fourteen years of service, it marked my bittersweet farewell to Highland Springs High School. Retirement was supposed to be a time of joyful reflection, but life had different plans. As years passed, my once-beloved school transformed. The air of learning and positivity I had worked so hard to nurture gave way to stress and disarray—a place marred by fights and the lingering scent of marijuana. The toll on my health was swift. As I drew closer to the school each morning, my blood pressure would rise. Stress crept into every corner of my life, and the health consequences were undeniable. Clinic visits became routine as the stress-fueled high blood pressure spiraled.

But it wasn't just my physical health. The weight on my heart was immense. I had built a nurturing environment for my students—a sanctuary where they could thrive. Watching it all unravel crushed me. Despite the toxic atmosphere, I pressed on, hoping for change.

I sought help. I spoke candidly with the Principal and Central Office, pouring my heart out in the hope they'd hear the cries for change. I even invited the superintendent to witness what we were living through daily. Her visit was a pivotal moment. As we walked the hallways together, the grim reality was impossible to ignore. She saw the grime and the tension in the air and listened as I shared my pain and frustrations. Her compassion provided a glimmer of hope.

But hope couldn't shield me from the relentless stress. No matter the efforts to improve conditions, the toll on my health was undeniable. It was time to choose myself. Retiring wasn't just about stepping away from work—it was about survival, finding peace, and reclaiming my health. Leaving behind a place I had poured so much into was heart-wrenching. The bonds with students, colleagues, and the community felt irreplaceable. But my health had to come first. I'd given everything, even at my own expense.

My final days were a mix of nostalgia and hope. Every hallway echoed memories—laughter, tears, milestones, and struggles. I said my goodbyes, cherishing every connection and every lesson learned. Retirement wasn't the end. It was a new beginning for me guided by God's purpose. My time at Highland Springs shaped me, leaving indelible lessons and cherished memories.

As I embraced retirement, I felt compelled to share my story. Teachers and students deserve safe, nurturing spaces to grow. My journey wasn't just mine—it was a call to action to spark change. And so, I moved forward with hope and faith, ready to continue making a difference. The chapter had changed, but the mission lived on, carried in my heart and actions with unwavering purpose.

Covid-2020 The Pandemic

Life is full of moments that reveal the divine timing of God—a reminder that while we may not always see the path ahead, there is a higher plan at work guiding us with care and purpose. This timing often feels miraculous, as if the pieces of our lives align perfectly when we need it most. It's a testament to trusting a force far more significant than ourselves.

To trust in divine timing means to hold faith that every challenge, twist, and triumph happens for a reason. Even when the journey feels uncertain, and our steps falter, there is comfort in knowing that every detour and delay is part of a more excellent plan. When we let go of worry and trust in this higher purpose, we find that life unfolds in ways more beautiful than we could ever imagine.

In 2020, the world stood still. The COVID-19 pandemic brought fear and turmoil, disrupting lives and routines and casting a shadow of uncertainty. Yet, amid the chaos, many of us discovered the power of surrendering to divine guidance. It was a time of challenge and awakening, where faith became a sanctuary and hope, a lifeline.

For me, this divine orchestration was undeniable. Just before the pandemic hit, I made the bittersweet decision to retire from Highland Springs High School. I could never have predicted the magnitude of what was to come, but God knew. Looking back, I see clearly how perfect His timing was. In those moments of doubt and grief over stepping away, I was shielded from the trials that would soon descend upon the world.

As schools became hotspots of uncertainty, I felt immense gratitude for the protection I had been granted. I witnessed God's timely provision—removing me from harm's way before the storm arrived. It was a humbling reminder of His care. While fear gripped the world, I leaned on faith. I prayed fervently for protection over my loved ones, singing the words that brought me strength:

"For my cleansing this I see—

Nothing but the Blood of Jesus.

This is all my hope and peace—

Nothing but the Blood of Jesus!"

These words carried me through the uncertainty. They reminded me that God's protection remained unshakable while the world shifted around us. I chose not to receive the COVID-19 vaccine, placing my faith instead in the shield of God's grace—and by His mercy, I remained untouched by the virus. My testimony became one of His steadfast faithfulness and strength, even in a world turned upside down.

The isolation brought by the pandemic invited deep reflection. Time spent at home became a sacred opportunity to draw closer to God. I immersed myself in prayer, studied His Word more intently, and strengthened my connection with Him. Even in solitude, I found community online, sharing prayers, stories, and strength with my church family. Together, we discovered that distance could never diminish our bonds or the light of faith.

Amid the uncertainty, I saw God's hand provide for every need—mine and others. Stories of healing, resilience, and unwavering faith multiplied each one a spark of hope. The pandemic, as devastating as it was, revealed the strength of the human spirit and the beauty of compassion, kindness, and divine guidance.

Through it all, I felt called to serve. I reached out with prayers and words of encouragement, sharing my story of God's miraculous timing and faithfulness. My mission became clear: to be a beacon of hope, reminding others that

God's light remains ever-present even in life's darkest valleys.

The lessons of 2020 endure. Life is fragile, but faith is unbreakable. God is our fortress, our unwavering source of strength in times of need. As we move forward, we do so with gratitude, purpose, and peace from trusting in His perfect plan. With God guiding our steps, every challenge can be met with courage, every struggle can transform into strength, and every ending can give way to a glorious new beginning.

21 Years Later

"Heal me, O Lord, and I shall be healed…" Jeremiah

17:14

"And he said unto me, my grace is sufficient for thee: my strength is perfect in weakness. Therefore, I will most gladly glory in my infirmities, that the power of Christ may rest upon me." – 2 Corinthians 12:9

Faith in God is a cornerstone of strength and hope, especially in adversity. Through faith, we find the courage to face life's challenges, knowing that we are never alone and that a higher power guides our journey. Faith can comfort us during the darkest moments, offering assurance that God is with us, always watching and leading.

But there are moments when faith alone may feel insufficient. Sometimes, our obstacles are so significant that we must seek help beyond ourselves from doctors, counselors, or other professionals. This is not a sign of weakness but rather an opportunity to recognize that God's guidance can come through these resources. By embracing help from others, we open ourselves to God's wisdom and remember that He works through all circumstances, providing us with the tools we need to heal.

Believing that God leads us to these earthly resources is, in itself, an act of faith. It shows trust in His wisdom and guidance, knowing He will direct us to the right people and places at the right time. Combining faith with the practical help available creates a powerful support system, enabling us to overcome life's challenges more effectively.

This truth became all too apparent after 21 years of relying on God's healing and guidance. My trust in God had helped me navigate many health issues, but in January 2023, I faced a new, unexpected struggle that tested my faith in ways I never anticipated.

It began with a sharp pain in my right abdomen, followed by persistent and severe nosebleeds. Each nosebleed felt like a warning that something was wrong. I prayed fervently, seeking God's intervention, but the silence was deafening. The pain worsened, and my body felt weak.

Then, two men of God (my brother and my Pastor) called me separately but on the same day, urging me to seek medical attention. They said, "Sister, you need to go get yourself checked, or you're going to die." Their words echoed in my mind, but I continued to pray, trusting that God would answer my cries for help.

On 23 January 2023, another severe nosebleed occurred while I was at my mother's house. My children's father worried about my health and insisted on taking me to the ER. As we drove, he expressed concern that it might be too late since I hadn't seen a doctor in over 20 years. His words pierced my heart, but I silently prayed as we made our way to the hospital.

At the emergency room, I was dizzy and disoriented. The nurse checked my blood pressure, which was dangerously high—200/91, at the stroke level. The doctors immediately began testing my heart, drawing blood, and running an EKG. They diagnosed me with hypertension and recommended medication, but I declined, saying, "No, thank you, I don't take medicine." I still trusted in God's healing.

By March 2023, I had lost 34 pounds. I visited the ER several more times due to a urinary tract infection and excruciating abdominal pain. My health was rapidly deteriorating. It was then that my pastor, seeing my condition, insisted that I seek medical attention. I was sick as unto to death, but as I lay on my sofa, I was resolved to die believing God. The spirit of God brought this scripture to me, 1 Corinthian 6:19-20: "What! Know you not that your body is the temple of the Holy Ghost which is in you, which you have of God, and ye are not your own? For ye are bought with a price: therefore, glorify God in your body and spirit, which are God's."

Reluctantly, I agreed to undergo a series of medical tests for the first time in almost two decades.

As someone who had not seen a doctor in years, my decision to seek medical care was difficult. However, I realized that turning to doctors did not diminish my trust in God. Instead, it showed that I was open to how He might bring healing and restoration into my life. I could seek help from modern medicine while maintaining my faith, confident that God's wisdom would guide me.

On 1 May 2023, I became eligible for Medicare. By 23 May, I turned 65 and chose a personal care physician who conducted a thorough checkup. The results revealed several health concerns, including an underactive thyroid. A pap smear and mammogram followed, and the mammogram showed a troubling spot in my left breast. A biopsy was ordered, and the diagnosis of invasive lobular carcinoma came soon after.

I was numb when I received the news: I had breast cancer. It was stage 3. The tumor was 15mm in diameter, and eight lymph nodes in the left axilla were infected. My heart sank, but I held firm in my faith, trusting that God had a plan for me, even in this moment of uncertainty.

Surgery was scheduled for 10 August 2023. When offered chemotherapy and medication, I chose to decline. I completely trusted God's plan, saying, "I am going to live until I die." I firmly believed that He would see me through this trial.

I agreed to take Radiation therapy only and it began soon after surgery and lasted for six weeks, concluding on 2 January 2024. I received exceptional care from the Massey Cancer Center at Stony Point during this time. The warmth and encouragement of my doctor and his staff were invaluable, lifting my spirits during the most challenging moments.

On the final day of my radiation treatment, I was invited to ring the bell, a symbol of completing this challenging treatment chapter. My family was there to witness the moment. They were always there for me. I felt an overwhelming sense of gratitude and victory as I rang the bell. My doctor later said he had never seen anyone ring the bell with such enthusiasm and joy.

This journey has been a testament to the power of prayer, faith, and the courage to accept help. It has been a journey of divine intervention, grace, and moments of profound strength. I have been reminded of God's presence, even in the most challenging times. And that God will place people in your life for "Such a time as this." People like my pastor and his wife. Thank you, Pastor!

Looking back, I am grateful for the strength God has given me. Despite the challenges, I remain confident in His plan for my life. This experience has deepened my faith, proving that with God, anything is possible. I continue to trust Him with my health, future, and very being, knowing He will always lead me toward healing and restoration.

Where I Am Today

"Therefore, I take pleasure in infirmities, reproaches, necessities, persecutions, distresses for Christ's sake: for when I am weak, then am I strong." – 2 Corinthians 12:10

Healing is a journey that demands inner strength and unwavering trust. For those who embark on it, the path is often strewn with challenges that test resilience and faith. Yet, faith—faith in God's plan—provides the courage to move forward. This belief in divine purpose offers solace, reminding us that even our pain has meaning. Through this lens of faith, we find the strength to endure and the conviction to press on.

Throughout healing, prayer and scripture become sanctuaries of peace and guidance. They are rituals and lifelines, grounding us in God's promises and love.

Immersing oneself in His Word grants wisdom and perspective, illuminating the path through pain and uncertainty. It reinforces the comforting truth that we are never alone—God is ever-present, guiding us with His unchanging hand.

As healing progresses, trust in God's plan deepens. Gradually, life begins to reflect the beauty of renewal, and the realization dawns that every challenge is part of a greater divine purpose. This understanding fosters profound gratitude and strengthens the relationship with God. Through this transformation, the healed become living testimonies of faith, inspiring others to trust in His plan and find strength in their journeys.

Reflecting on the past year, my heart overflows with gratitude. A year ago, I was in a dark place, overwhelmed by pain, fear, and anxiety. But God, in His infinite love and grace, walked with me through every trial. He never left my side. He sent people—prayer warriors—who stood in faith for my healing. My pastor, persistent despite my resistance, often said, "You're a hard nut to crack," but he never gave up on me.

Before undergoing surgery, I fervently prayed for God to guide my doctor's hands, trusting the Great Physician to work through him. After the procedure, my doctor said my prayers had profoundly moved him, filling him with a sense of humility and responsibility. This reaffirmed what I already knew—God was in control, orchestrating my healing through the medical team's expertise He had placed in my life.

The journey of recovery has been one of faith and perseverance. Today, I can say with joy that I am healing beautifully. The burning and peeling, once akin to a relentless sunburn, have significantly diminished. The surgical site, encompassing my left breast and underarm, is steadily improving, each day a testament to God's healing power.

Soon, I'll undergo a mammogram to confirm that the cancer is gone and ensure I'm firmly on the road to full recovery. I approach this step with confidence, trusting that the results will affirm my progress and further validate the faithfulness of God's promises.

This process taught me to lean on God more deeply than ever before. Psalm 46:1 reminds us that He is "our refuge and strength, an ever-present help in trouble." My faith has been both tested and fortified. I've come to understand that healing is not just a physical process but a profound spiritual journey.

This past year has also been a time of reflection and growth. Looking back, I see how God has worked in every aspect of my life. From the moment I heard His voice declare my healing to the challenges of navigating cancer treatment without traditional interventions, each experience has been a chapter in the story of His faithfulness.

One of the most valuable lessons I've learned is the power of gratitude. Even in moments of hardship and uncertainty, there is always something to be thankful for— the unwavering support of my family, my church community's prayers, and my medical team's dedication. Above all, I am grateful for God's unfailing love and presence.

As I continue to heal, I feel compelled to share my story. I pray that others will see the light of Christ in my journey and understand that they, too, can find hope and healing in Him. My journey is far from over, but I trust that God will continue to guide me, using my testimony for His glory.

Looking to the future, I am filled with hope and anticipation. While I know there will be challenges ahead, I also know that the God who has carried me this far will not abandon me. He has a plan for my life that is greater than I can imagine, and I am excited to see it unfold.

In summary, this past year has been a journey of transformation and renewal. From the depths of despair to the heights of faith, I have experienced God's healing touch in every aspect of my life. Today, I stand as a living testament to His mercy and grace. With a grateful heart and steadfast faith, I move forward, knowing that God's purpose for my life is still being written.

Thank You, Lord, for bringing me such a long way. I will forever praise Your name and proclaim Your goodness. Amen.

Cancer Free

On 1 August 2024, my mammogram was scheduled for 10:00 a.m. My breast imaging exam results were nothing short of miraculous: expected. My mammogram revealed that my breast tissue was not dense, and there was no evidence of anything concerning. My follow-up recommendation is a 3D Diagnostic Mammogram in one year—scheduled for 2 August 2025.

What a blessing! What a relief! I thank God!

My cancer had been diagnosed at Stage 3—a daunting reality. Yet here I was, cancer-free. I thank God for this miracle!

I made unconventional choices during my treatment journey. I declined chemotherapy and chose radiation instead. I also refused the estrogen pill. These decisions were not easy, and

I made them prayerfully, leaning on my faith every step of the way. God's grace has carried me through, and I stand as a living testament to His healing power.

To God be the Glory! I am a Miracle!

www.ingramcontent.com/pod-product-compliance
Lightning Source LLC
Chambersburg PA
CBHW051240120626
46547CB00014B/1729